# Opening Reflection

## Personal Reflection from the Creator of the Cerebro-Vital Support System (CVSS)

For those who find this work after me.

I didn't set out to save the world. I didn't even set out to change it.

In the beginning, the Cerebro-Vital Support System wasn't a solution to anything. It was just a question:

"What if we didn't have to let the mind die just because the body failed?"

That was it. A single, disquieting thought I couldn't shake.

I didn't imagine it would grow. That it would pull me into this vast, lonely architecture of possibilities. That it would become something capable of replacing every function of the human body. That it would force me to wrestle with life, death, identity, autonomy—everything we think makes us human.

But it did.

And the deeper I went, the more I realized what I had truly stumbled into:

This isn't just a machine. This is a doorway.

Not to immortality, not to perfection. But to continuity. To choice.

A way for human consciousness to keep going when biology says "no more."

I've spent countless nights working alone. I've watched the sun rise and fall over a world seemingly hopeless in it's current state. Wondering if anyone would ever understand what this system I've envisioned truly is. Not a rebellion against nature. Not an affront to life. But a tribute to it.

A preservation of its most sacred element: the mind that dreams.

If you're reading this—if you've found the AegisARC framework and you're continuing its path—then maybe I wasn't alone after all. Maybe...it just wasn't time yet.

You may feel what I have felt: isolation, doubt, even fear. The world resists change. Institutions resist independence. And some will do everything they can to preserve the old systems of control.

But stay steady.

You are not building a device.
You are building a right.


The right to think. The right to remain. The right to be—even when the flesh says you shouldn't.

So here, to you, I leave what I could not finish.
Not a legacy. Not a monument. Just the first piece in a bridge I
was never meant to cross alone.

Keep going.
And may your mind never be silenced.

–The Architect Unnamed
Originator CVSS | AegisARC

# Prologue

The human, the product of millions of years of evolution—an intricate, beautiful accident of survival rather than a deliberate design for longevity. Beneath our skin lies a fragile code stitched by chance—cells programmed for decay, organs susceptible to disease and trauma, a ship ill equipped for the voyage. Our bones calcify, our cells mutate, our muscle and joints grow weak—and yet we are told to see this deterioration as natural, even beautiful. But what is beautiful about helplessness? Our species, so bold in its conquests of land and sky, is shackled to a form that surrenders daily to entropy.

Throughout history, humanity has fought against this entropy. From the earliest herbal medicines to modern organ transplants, we have been at war with our own biology. Yet even our most advanced interventions have merely delayed the inevitable. The plagues of the Middle Ages, the influenza pandemic of 1918, the ongoing battles against cancer and neurodegenerative diseases— each reminds us that biology is not a fortress but a crumbling wall. Every year, despite billions spent on healthcare, millions die of conditions rooted in the body's natural collapse.

But it is not only the body that fails. It is the systems we built around it.

Civilizations grow like organisms: expanding, consuming, aging. And just like organisms, they falter when overstretched. The fall of Rome was not a singular catastrophe, but a slow erosion of resources, governance, and resilience. Today, the signs of systemic exhaustion are global. We teeter on the edge of a population tipping point, with resources dwindling and infrastructures buckling under the weight of demand. Global freshwater supplies are strained. Arable land shrinks under the press of cities and climate change. Economic inequality deepens, healthcare systems collapse under the burden of the terminal, and families watch loved ones fade, not for lack of love, but for lack of time, space, and molecular luck.

Just as our bodies are limited by cellular decay, so too are our institutions limited by short-term thinking, finite energy, and aging infrastructure. Without intervention, both biological and civilization collapse are inevitable, linked by the same failure to adapt beyond old frameworks.

We've built machines to carry us. Drugs to numb us. Networks to connect us. Yet the body remains the bottleneck.

Advancements in robotics, artificial intelligence, and biotechnology have given humanity tools unimaginable even a century ago. Yet our dominant paradigm still chains consciousness to a decaying chassis of flesh. We extend life by years, but not vitality. We add decades to human existence, but too often those years are spent in frailty, pain, or cognitive decline. Predictions from institutions like the United Nations and WHO suggest that by 2050, the number of people over 60 will double—an aging population straining already fragile systems to the breaking point. Without trans-formative intervention, humanity faces an era of mass geriatric dependency, environmental collapse, and societal fragmentation.

In care homes across the world, minds remain sharp while bodies collapse in place—trapped in beds, waiting for the body's permission to die. Each silent room, each forgotten story, is a testament to what happens when biology outlives its utility but not its suffering.

And so the question arises, what if the body is no longer the solution, but the problem? This is not a question born from arrogance, but necessity. What if we were able to relegate chronic disease, paralysis, natural aging and even death from bodily failure to the history books. The day has come where science and technology can allow us to achieve these lofty goals.

The system, known in development as the Cerebro-Vital Support System (CVSS), and publicly as AegisARC. It is a combination of synthetic systems that replace all the biological functions of the human body below the neck. An array of mechanisms and technology developed to mimic all of the organs and processes that sustain the brain. It utilizing a design philosophy to be more durable, sustainable and upgradable than biology.
A system not born not in rebellion of biology, but in recognition: that the mind is sacred, and the body is expendable. This is not science fiction. The architecture contained here is rooted in real tangible systems combined to act as bridge for humanity to pass into a new chapter of existence. This is not a rejection of humanity. It is a defense of it.

This book is intended to be a record, a guide, and a declaration for those who feel the tremors beneath our feet and know that tomorrow must be different—not by decree, but by intelligent and responsible design.

Let this be the beginning of that design—one that remembers who we are, while redefining what we can become.

# Part I: The Problem of Continuance

## Cultural Fear of Death vs. Fear of Change

Much of society has grown comfortable with death because it fears the alternative: uncertainty. To consider outliving the body is to confront a philosophical abyss. What are we without our skin? Without our breath? Without the rituals of finality we have built entire civilizations around? The answer to these questions is you will still be you. Human consciousness is contained in the cerebral cortex. That astoundingly complex three pound array of gray matter in your skull is you.

Fear of death has been mythologized, ritualized, and domesticated. From ancient Egypt's elaborate funerary cults to modern bioethics debates, humanity has repeatedly shown a preference for the known darkness over the unknown dawn. This is because the fear of change is more potent, more real, more paralyzing. We have taught ourselves to mourn death, but we have never taught ourselves how to survive transformation.

This fear blinds us to opportunity. In clinging to the familiar, we deny the possibility of liberation—not only from disease, but from limitation itself.

Every great societal leap—whether the abolition of slavery, the rise of women's rights, or the acceptance of space exploration—was first met with terror that "changing the natural order" would lead to chaos.

And yet, change is the only true constant of existence.

If we continue to worship death as a necessary end, we will close the door to the most ethical evolution of all: the continuance of conscious life beyond biological decay.

## Medical Systems as Maintenance, Not Liberation

Medicine, as we know it, is largely palliative. It postpones. It treats symptoms. It manages decline.

Billions are spent each year to maintain failing biological systems a little longer—systems already structurally doomed to collapse.

Historical examples abound:

In the 20th century, polio wards filled with iron lungs preserved breath but not vitality.

In the 21st century, we see ICUs where life is extended mechanically without restoring agency or dignity.

We congratulate ourselves for heroic measures that extend life by weeks or months, yet we do not question whether the scaffold is worth saving at all.

Imagine a building project that utilized exorbitant amounts of time, money and resources to build a bridge that ultimately leads to nowhere. At the end of the road there is nothing more than a giant abyss ready to swallow all who travel.

We repair failing bodies without daring to ask whether the model of "body-first" medicine is itself obsolete.

True medicine should not merely extend the timeline of suffering.

It should liberate life from the prison of structural failure. It should protect consciousness—not the vehicle it happens to inhabit. If your car was broken down would you simply accept this, give up, and never go anywhere ever again? Of course not, its not in our nature. You would simply find a different means of transport.

To maintain without liberating is not compassion. It is complicity.

## Technological Paralysis and the Ethics of Delay

We possess the knowledge.

We possess the means.

But we delay.

We delay because of fear: fear of backlash, fear of disruption, fear of unintended consequences.

The scientific consensus on anesthesia existed decades before it was accepted into surgical practice.

The basic principles of germ theory were known, yet hand washing was resisted by physicians for decades at the cost of countless lives.

In our own era, gene therapy and regenerative technologies are shackled not by technical failure, but by bureaucratic, legal, and cultural hesitation.

We delay because of power: entrenched interests that profit from managing decay rather than curing it.

The powers that control and manipulate society for thier own personal satisfaction would greatly fear this change. It is no fault of their own. We should hold no ill will against politicians and corporations. They are only doing what evolution has taught them. The inability to be selfless when in power comes from our minds evolving and living in a scarcity environment. Our ape brain tells us to survive we need to hoard resources, smash opponents, do what every we must. This is why our political systems still don't work. If you give a primate the means to control all aspects of its survival and contentment it would hold onto that power until its last breath.

So the AegisARC is not only a biological transformation and rebirth but also a cultural one. A harbinger new beginnings. Our systems of government and control would need to pledge above all else to remain ethical and selfless to guide humanity into a new age. To never capitalize or profit from an individuals right to choose life. And to vehemently oppose any efforts to extort, exploit or exclude any person.

We delay because of tradition: a psychological inertia that values the familiar corpse over the unfamiliar continuum. But to fear and delay is in itself unethical. Every year we wait, millions suffer needlessly. Families lose loved ones not because death was unavoidable, but because societal inertia outweighed ethical urgency.

Ethical progress demands not hesitation, but courage. The longer we delay the redesign of life, the more complicit we become in the avoidable suffering we refuse to address. If we continue to cling to obsolete systems—whether biological or societal—we deny ourselves the next phase of human evolution

The question is no longer whether we can sustain human consciousness beyond biology.

It is whether we have the moral clarity to admit that we must.

We will never see the light of a new sunrise if we continue to cower in our caves.

# Part II: The Case for CVSS and Post-Humanism

## Origins of the Concept

The Cerebro-Vital Support System (CVSS) did not emerge from a laboratory funded by corporate futurism or from a committee of technocrats.

It began as a question—posed by one person, alone in the quiet discomfort of awareness:

From that seed grew a design that sought not to defeat death, but to remove its most arbitrary cause: the failure of the vessel.

History has often pivoted on such solitary questions.

Galileo asked why Earth must be the center of everything.

Darwin asked whether species could change.

Alan Turing asked whether machines could think.

Each of these questions destabilized centuries of certainty. Each was met with resistance, ridicule—and ultimately, transformation.

CVSS was born from the same lineage of inquiry: not from hubris, conquest or control, but a humble recognition that our reverence for biology must not become a prison.

In an era obsessed with extending wealth rather than wisdom, the idea of extending thought itself—free from biological constraint—remains revolutionary.

## Design as Philosophy: Why Support the Brain

In choosing to sustain only the brain and its immediate biological interfaces, CVSS draws a deliberate line of functionality:

**Everything below is replaceable; everything above is sacred.**

This is not trans-humanism in its sensationalist form.
It is not the uploading of consciousness into cold digital replicas.

It is not the fabrication of identity in silicon. It is **continuance without compromise**.

The brain remains human. The support becomes synthetic.
Modern neuroscience confirms that our sense of identity—our memories, emotions, consciousness—resides in specific, delicate structures of the brain.

It is not our hands or our legs that make us who we are; it is the hippocampus that stores memory, the prefrontal cortex that contemplates ethics, the amygdala that loves and fears.
We already accept technological augmentation without question: pacemakers, ventilators, dialysis machines.

CVSS is simply the next logical step—a natural extension of medical technology toward the preservation of consciousness itself.

If medical technology were a living organism, CVSS would be its evolutionary flowering.

In an age rushing toward artificial intelligence and machine replication, the CVSS stands as a testament:

**That the biological brain—the dreaming, suffering, loving human brain—is still the irreplaceable cathedral of consciousness.**

## The Ethics of Continuance

To continue is not to escape morality, but to **fulfill it**.
CVSS is built on the principle that every person deserves the chance to persist—to sustain their mind until it is no longer viable by natural degeneration, not arbitrary bodily failure.

That choice—the right to extend consciousness—must not be reserved for the wealthy, the powerful, or the privileged.
It must be protected, decentralized, and universally accessible.

Continuity must never become a commodity.

History teaches us the risks of technological inequality.

During the Industrial Revolution, advances in mechanization benefited the few at the cost of the many.

During the rise of computing, access was initially a privilege of the elite.

Without foresight and ethical governance, every great leap forward has threatened to widen the chasm between the empowered and the powerless.

We must ensure that CVSS does not follow this path.
Those who adopt this next stage of existence must never forget their humanity.

The underlying principle must remain unchanged: **we are one species, coexisting on the only viable planet we currently have.**

The true measure of success will not be the number of lives extended.

It will be the dignity with which those lives are honored—whether biological, synthetic, or something new entirely.

Continuity without equity is not progress.
It is dystopia.

## How CVSS Could Change Everything

If adopted at scale, CVSS could relieve global health systems of their crushing burdens.

It could reduce human reliance on food production, agricultural exploitation, and finite medical resources—thereby reducing environmental strain.

It could extend productive intellectual life beyond the arbitrary limitations of physical decline. By providing a stable, controlled, biologically ideal environment the human brain may plausibly persist far beyond its current lifespan. Perhaps 120-200 years, theoretically.

Imagine teachers imparting wisdom across centuries.
Imagine artists evolving their styles over lifetimes unconstrained by aging flesh.

Imagine scientists not bound by the biological clock, but by the depth of their curiosity.

It redefines the aging process.

It reframes the idea of disability—not as a deficiency to be pitied, but as a set of challenges with technological solutions.
It transforms what it means to medically "treat" a person—from restoring a broken body to protecting an evolving mind.
Most importantly, it opens a door to a future where **survival is no longer measured by skin, but by mind**.

But this gift brings responsibilities:

- Psychological endurance for potentially centuries-long consciousness.
- Ethical models for governance when leaders may no longer die in office.
- New understandings of risk, creativity, boredom, renewal.
-

We must prepare ourselves not only for extended survival —but for the flourishing of the mind across unimaginable spans of time.

When survival is no longer limited by the durability of flesh, **the mind is finally liberated to pursue knowledge, empathy, and discovery on a scale our ancestors could never have dreamed.**

# Part III: Short Stories from the Future

## The First Continuant

Selene awoke to stillness.

Not the stillness of sleep, nor the restless silence of illness.

A deeper stillness — a silence within herself.

No heartbeat. No breath.

And yet she was not dead.

Her mind flickered into clarity, raw and immediate. Memories surged: the hospital bed, the whispered goodbyes, the failing heart monitors. She remembered the pain, the struggle, the steady erosion of her body's loyalty.

And she remembered the choice.

The last choice she had made — against fear, against certainty.

A choice not to surrender.

A choice to continue.

Selene tried to move. There was weight — gravity still tethered her — but her muscles did not respond in the old way. Instead, a smooth, coordinated shifting of balance occurred. Her awareness stretched outward, discovering sensation anew: the texture of synthetic proprioception humming gently through her.

It was not numbness. It was... different.

A body, rebuilt not in flesh, but in function.

She opened her eyes. The room was small, white, clean. A soft mechanical hum vibrated the air, steady and reassuring. A wall of glass separated her from a small cluster of observers — five figures in sterile suits, faces earnest but restrained, holding their breath as if one sound might break the fragile miracle unfolding before them.

One stepped forward — a woman, perhaps mid-forties, her gloved hand trembling slightly as she touched a control panel. The glass partition dissolved into transparency.

She spoke.

"You made it," she said, voice breaking at the edges.

"You're the first."

Selene blinked. Her eyes slightly dry. She could still her the low buzzing of her tinitus. But there was a new sound, quiet and low coming from her chest.
The systems now supporting her life. Systems replacing what the body had once done without thought.

She found her voice — fragile, yet unmistakably her own.

"I'm..."

She paused, feeling the word resonate somewhere deep inside. "I'm still here."

Tears blurred her vision. Her — still her — tears.

The woman on the other side of the glass wiped her own eyes hastily, stepping back to give Selene space. No applause. No celebration. Only reverence.
Selene reached up instinctively and touched the back of her neck. Beneath the synthetic skin interface, she could feel the ridges of the C3 Collar — the interface with her remaining biological core. At her temples, she felt the light mesh of the Supplemental Sensors, reading her cortical fields.

Beyond that — nothing.

No heartbeat.

No lungs expanding.

No muscle ache.

Only the whisper of the CVSS — the Cerebro-Vital Support System — sustaining her.

And her mind — untouched. Her memories intact. Her soul, whatever it was, still unmistakably hers.

Selene closed her eyes. In that darkness, she waited for the fear to rise — the existential terror that every philosopher had warned of, the despair of losing the body, the grief of becoming something other.

But the fear never came.
Instead, she felt... gratitude. A solemn, vast gratitude — not for the machine, not even for the survival itself — but for the preservation of what mattered.
Her mind, her memories, her hope.

She thought of her family — some who had understood, some who had begged her not to go through with it.

She thought of the world she had left — crumbling infrastructures, aging populations, the quiet, growing desperation that clung to hospitals and homes alike.

And she thought of the future — unwritten, uncertain, but now open to her.

Slowly, Selene stood. The CVSS responded perfectly, compensating for the shift of balance, maintaining circulation, thermoregulation, sensory input.

Every movement was deliberate. Every moment was real.

She walked — carefully, but easily — toward the glass.
The caretakers stepped back, allowing her the dignity of those first steps in this new existence.
Beyond them, through the larger windows, she could see the sunrise cresting the horizon.

The world she had known. The world she still belonged to.

Selene placed her hand against the cool surface of the glass and whispered:

"This is not a rebirth. It's a keeping."

The words fell into the silence like a vow.

Not a rejection of humanity. Not an abandonment of her self. A continuation.

The CVSS was not her captor. It was her steward.
It was the bridge she had chosen to cross, past the river of flesh and into something new.

Selene turned back toward the small team watching her, their expressions a mixture of awe and responsibility.

"I will not waste this," she said softly.
And in that moment — in that quiet, defiant oath — she became not just the first Continuant.
She became a keeper of the future.

# The Silent Decade

The memorial center was almost empty.

Elias stood awkwardly near the edge of the polished
floor, hands clasped in front of him, staring at the
simple holo-display.

It showed a women's face — calm, smiling, alive.
Not a tombstone. Not a memorial of death.
A tribute to continuance.

His mother had chosen the CVSS transition two
months earlier. Quietly. Without ceremony. Without
even telling many of the family. She had called it her
"second sunrise."

But to most of the world, it was still seen as something
else entirely: a betrayal.

Around him, the room echoed with silence. A few
chairs stood empty. A few flowers had been left in
confusion, unsure whether they honored life or mocked
it.

Outside the center, a small group had gathered —
protesters holding signs.

"Defilers of Life!"

"Only God Decides!"

"Continuants Are Not Human!"

Elias lowered his gaze. He had known this would happen. The fear campaigns had done their work well. The news outlets had been relentless: headlines screaming about soulless machines, the death of humanity, the elite stealing eternity from the common man.

Governments had stalled certification processes. Religious authorities had thundered from pulpits about abominations.

Whisper networks had spread dystopian horror stories faster than any truth could travel.
For ten years after the first Continuants — after Selene — society had recoiled.

CVSS adoption froze. Facilities closed. Scientists were blacklisted. Families were divided.
It was called the Silent Decade. A decade of waiting.
A decade of fear.

Elias clenched his fists. His own siblings had refused to come today. His aunts and uncles had stopped speaking to him after his mother's transition.

In their eyes, she had died anyway.
Better to have perished naturally than to step into the unknown.

And yet, here he stood. Because he had heard her voice. He had listened, weeks after her procedure, as she spoke from her recovery room.
Her laughter, her thoughts, her mind — fully herself.
Preserved. Continuing.

He stepped forward now, closer to the simple pedestal where her holo stood. A small speaker embedded in the frame clicked gently to life.

"Thank you," her voice said, strong and clear.

"For believing that life is more than breath alone."

Elias swallowed hard. A lump caught in his throat.
"I know this is not what you imagined," she continued.
"I know the world is afraid. But fear is not a verdict. It is only a threshold."

Outside, the protests grew louder. A chant rising. A crude song filled with anger and desperation.
Elias closed his eyes.

Was it wrong to defy death? Was it arrogant to extend a life when nature said otherwise? Was it selfish to want to hear her voice still, to know she was not lost?

He opened his eyes again and saw, not just his mother's face, but something larger.

The dignity of choice. The defiance of despair.

It was not arrogance. It was courage. And the fear outside was not proof of wrongdoing. It was proof that something new had been born — and the old world was mourning its own coming obsolescence.

Elias placed his hand gently against the base of the holo-display. It was warm. Alive in its own way.

He whispered, barely audible over the growing clamor beyond the glass:

"I will not let them shame this."

Outside, someone pounded against the center doors.

Inside, the light of the display held steady. A symbol, small but unbroken.

Elias turned, walking through the vestibule and out into the courtyard.

The protesters jeered as he emerged, pushing signs toward him, shouting words meant to wound.
But he kept walking, slow and steady.

Because he understood now. Continuance would not be won by argument. It would not be won by violence. It would endure the way all true revolutions endure: quietly, patiently, irrevocably.

The Silent Decade would pass. Fear would break against the unchanging presence of those who had chosen to remain.

And when it did — when humanity found the courage to look beyond the fear — they would find that the future had been waiting for them all along.
Waiting with a heartbeat not of flesh, but of memory.

Waiting with arms not of bone, but of will.
Waiting, with minds that had refused to be forgotten.

## Children of the Second Sun

The sun slanted low across the hills, bathing the world in gold.

Aiden lay in the tall grass, kicking his bare feet against the soil, a crumpled datapad beside him.
Above, a lone hawk circled in the deepening blue.
The breeze was warm against his skin. The earth was warm under his body.

It all felt... normal. Ordinary. Until he remembered.

Not far away, standing at the edge of the field, his mother waited. Motionless, serene — her frame wrapped in the light, the subtle hum of her CVSS just audible in the quiet afternoon.

To anyone who didn't know, she looked almost ordinary: human silhouette, natural posture, even everyday clothing for ease of social interaction.

But Aiden knew. Everyone knew.

Continuants were not like the others.
He sat up, hugging his knees, feeling the old anger spark in his chest.

Earlier that day, at school, he had heard the words again. Whispers. Laughs.

"Ghost child."

"Your mom is a dead thing pretending."

"You're not even real."

He hadn't fought back. Not with fists. Just silent resilience. But the words still scraped raw behind his ribs.

Now, in the golden quiet, he found himself staring at the one person who had anchored his life — and questioning it all.

"Why didn't you just..."

He hesitated, chewing the inside of his cheek.
His mother turned slightly, her now enhanced hearing undoubtedly registering the change in his tone.
"Why didn't you just let go?" Aiden said finally, the words tumbling out bitter.

"Everyone else's parents... they lived, they died. They moved on."

A long silence stretched between them.
Only the wind moved, whispering through the grass.
At last, his mother walked slowly toward him — each step deliberate, precise. Not mechanical. Just careful.

She knelt in the grass beside him, the synthetic dermal layers catching the light with an almost imperceptible sheen.

When she spoke, her voice was warm — not the hollow mimicry the children at school imagined, but vibrant, unmistakably human.

"I didn't stay because I feared death," she said quietly.

"I stayed because I loved you."

Aiden swallowed hard, looking away.

She continued:

"I made a promise, the day you were born. To protect you. To guide you. To stand by you — not until my body failed, but for as long as I could choose it."

Her hand reached out — not forcing, not demanding — simply offering.

After a long moment, Aiden took it. The synthetic hand
was warm. Steady. Alive. Tears pricked the corners of
his eyes.

"I don't want you to be a freak," he whispered. "I don't
want to be a freak."

Her fingers tightened gently around his.

"You are not a freak, Aiden.

You are a boy. A boy with a mother who love you.
You are not less and neither am I."

He pressed his forehead against their shoulder, feeling
the faint hum of the synthetic systems working
beneath.
Not cold. Not hollow. Alive.

After a while, they stood together, the field stretching
endless around them.

In the weeks that followed, something in Aiden shifted.
When another Continuant child — a girl whose father
had transitioned — was cornered behind the
schoolhouse, Aiden stepped in.

Not with aggression. Just presence. Just refusal.

"No more", he shouted.

It was not a grand rebellion.It was a beginning.

Aiden learned to walk with his head high, even when the whispers followed. He learned to love the moments that mattered, not the shells they came wrapped in.

And at night, he would look up at the stars and wonder: Which world did he truly belong to?

The first — the biological inheritance of blood and breath?
Or the second — the chosen light of preservation, of continuance, of unbroken memory?

Maybe both. Maybe neither. Maybe something new altogether.

He smiled into the night sky, the vast future arching above him. A child of two worlds.

And a world not yet ready for him — but coming. Slowly. Inevitably.

## The Betrayal of Flesh

A meeting of world leaders had been called to discuss the "conitinuant problem". The grand chamber was heavy with the scent of polished wood and aging power.

High above, stained-glass skylights cast fractured light across the debating floor, illuminating faces twisted by fear, greed, and something older still — the hunger to control.

Noah waited in silence at the edge of the proceedings, his synthetic frame cloaked beneath a simple robe, indistinguishable at a glance from the biological delegates that filled the hall.

Only those who knew where to look — the subtle perfection of his balance, the absence of involuntary movements — would recognize him as a Continuant.

The irony was bitter. He had been invited. But not to participate. Only to observe — like an artifact, a specimen.
The central dais glowed as Chancellor Morrow, voice sharp as cracked ice, pounded the lectern.

"We must act!" she thundered.

"We must recognize the existential threat these Continuants represent! If life is no longer bound to death, if allegiance to flesh is abandoned, then what separates humanity from its own extinction?"

Murmurs of agreement rippled through the chamber.

Here and there, banners fluttered — old nations, old faiths, old fears reborn under new names.

Noah watched without expression as the proposals were laid bare. Mandatory licensing for all Continuants. Asset seizures from those who transitioned without state approval. Banishment from political office. Denial of inheritance rights.
The slow erasure of citizenship. And, behind closed doors — whispered negotiations for patents.

The corporations eager to divide the CVSS designs among themselves, to carve up human continuance as a new frontier for profit.
They did not fear Continuants because they misunderstood them. They feared them because they could not own them.

Noah stood when his name was called — a procedural courtesy, nothing more. The hall fell uncomfortably silent. He stepped forward, the footsteps of his synthetic frame resonating against the stone, echoing throughout the chamber.

"I was not invited to speak," he said, his voice even, amplified across the room.

"But I will."

Morrow scowled, rising halfway from her chair — but something in Noah's presence held her back.
He turned slowly, addressing the room — and, beyond it, into the cameras, the millions watching from their homes in glass towers amid crumbling cities.

"I am not here to debate whether Continuants are human," he said.

"I am not here to beg for rights that are mine by existence alone."
He paused, letting the words settle.

"I am here to remind you," he said, "that the betrayal is not Continuance."

He scanned their faces — some flushed with anger, some pale with fear.

"The betrayal is flesh without compassion. Governance without dignity. Power without purpose."

A murmur of protest began to rise, but he pressed on, voice cutting through like a blade.

"You fear Continuance because you fear a humanity you cannot chain to suffering. You fear a humanity that remembers choice. That reclaims its right to dream without decay."

He let the silence stretch then, offering no comfort.

"You do not worship life," he said softly.

"You worship control. But you do not control me."

The chairwoman banged her gavel, calling for security. Noah smiled faintly. They could not arrest what they could not contain. With deliberate calm, he stepped back, turned, and walked peacefully out of the hall.

Behind him, the machinery of fear ground on, passing edicts and pronouncements against an inevitability they could neither halt nor truly comprehend.

That night, beneath the fractured glow of the city's edge, Noah entered a Continuant enclave — a hidden network pulsing quietly below the surveillance grids.

There, in a room softly lit only by data screens, he recorded a message. Not a call to arms. Not a threat. A remembrance.

"We are not deviations. We are not monsters.
We are not errors of ambition nor blasphemies of pride.
We are the stewards of what you have forgotten to cherish: The sovereignty of self"

He closed the file, encrypted it, and sent it into the networks — a seed waiting for the right time to bloom.

The world would rage. The governments would tighten their fists. The corporations would scheme.
But the dream of Continuance could not be revoked.
It was already alive — moving silently through hearts and minds that had not yet found the courage to speak.

And when the old world finally collapsed beneath the weight of its own fear, the Continuants would be there — not to conquer, not to avenge — but to remember what had been forgotten.

The simple, eternal dignity of life chosen freely.

## The Pilgrims

The launch fields stretched to the horizon — silver ships gleaming like rippling waves.
Mae stood at the edge of the gathering, her gaze tracing the arcs of scaffolding, the last work crews pulling away cables, sealing hatches.

The ships were small compared to the old dreams of colonization — no need for biological farms, cryogenic tanks, endless provisions. Continuants did not require what flesh demanded. They needed only memory. Mind. And time.

The sky above a deep violet, the first stars already seeding the dusk. A knot of people clustered near the base of the nearest vessel — families, friends, strangers. Some biological, some Continuant.
Some saying farewell with tears. Some with prayers. Some with accusations.

"You're abandoning us," a man shouted across the clearing, voice raw. "You think you're better than us!"

Mae said nothing. She had heard it before.
Continuants were no longer protected by myth.

They were real now — visible, tangible — and that frightened the old order more than any imagined crime.

They were proof that flesh was not the only road. Proof that existence could evolve without permission.

Mae adjusted the simple tunic she wore, an old habit of lingering modesty. There was still a part of her that longed to pass unnoticed among the biological crowds. But that life was gone. By choice. By design. She had chosen this.

Still, a heaviness clung to her as she turned back toward the embarkation platforms.
Memory weighed more than any synthetic body ever could.

She wandered the edge of the gathering, letting her mind drift through old streets. The schoolhouse where she had learned to read. The small garden where she had married her late husband. The quiet, crumbling library where she had once dreamed of the stars. Every memory, vivid. Every sensation intact.
Continuance had preserved her mind — but memory did not always ease the grief of departure.

She paused near a supply tent, watching a group of children chasing one another through the dust.

Their laughter drifting into the night. One boy — no older than seven — saw her standing apart.

He broke from the others, shyly approaching.
In his small hand, he held a carving — a rough little bird whittled from wood, wings outstretched as if caught midflight. Wordlessly, he offered it to her.

Mae knelt, taking the gift carefully in her hands.
The wood was warm from his fingers. The carving crude but beautiful — a simple gesture: to create, to give, to connect.

She met the boy's gaze — bright, fearless.

"What's its name?" she asked, her voice steady, low.

He shrugged.

"You can name it," he said.

Mae smiled — a small, trembling thing.
She rose slowly, tucking the bird carefully against her chest.

"Thank you," she whispered.

The boy beamed and ran back toward his companions, swallowed again by the twilight.

Mae stood for a long moment, cradling the carved bird.

When the signal came — a soft harmonic pulse resonating through the air — the Continuants gathered without fanfare. There were no speeches.
No anthems. No final declarations.

They had already spoken with their lives. They had already chosen.

The ships opened like unfolding petals, welcoming them aboard.

Mae climbed the ramp slowly, savoring each step — not because she regretted, but because she honored.
At the threshold, she turned one last time, looking out across the launch fields, the hills, the dim glow of the city beyond.
Earth would go on. Biological humanity would continue, with all its grief and brilliance and contradiction. And so would they — the Continuants — not as conquerors, not as deserters, but as stewards. Carrying forward the dream that had first lifted their ancestors from the plains, from the oceans, from the gravity wells of fear.

The dream to endure. To reach. To become.

Inside the vessel, Mae placed the wooden bird beside the navigation console. A compass to guide her. Not of circuits, but of memory.

The vessel lifted, silent and smooth, joining the others in slow ascent. From the ground, they looked like meteors reversed — not falling, but rising, pulling the future upward with them.

Mae closed her eyes, feeling the gentle pulse of synthetic blood through her preserved brain.
No fear. Only wonder.

They were the Pilgrims. Not fleeing death. Not abandoning humanity. Becoming its next verse — sung in the dark between the stars.

# Part IV: The Treatise on Continuance

## Preamble

We, the inheritors of a world shaped by mortality, suffering, and the limits of biology, now stand at the threshold of transformation. The Cerebro-Vital Support System (CVSS) — known as AegisARC — represents not the conquest of death, but the conscious choice to extend life with dignity.

This technology is not a product, but a philosophy: that every conscious being has the right to choose their continuity, to sustain identity free from coercion, commodification, or institutional control.

We present this Ethical Treatise to preserve the soul of this transition, and to declare that:

## Ten Core Ethical Principles

1.  Sovereignty of Consciousness: The right to exist, continue, or pass on shall remain with the individual—not with any government, corporation, or collective.

2.  Voluntary Transition: No individual shall be compelled, coerced, or manipulated into synthetic continuation. AegisARC shall always require conscious, informed consent.

3. Freedom from Ownership: The CVSS shall not be owned, patented, or monopolized. Its foundational architecture shall remain open, decentralized, and universally accessible.

4. Equitable Access: The right to synthetic life support shall not be contingent on wealth, citizenship, or privilege. The technology must be developed with equity at its core.

5. Transparency and Audit-ability: All source protocols, hardware schematics, and bio-synthetic standards must be transparent, reviewable, and free from proprietary obfuscation.

6. No Weaponization: AegisARC shall never be used as a weapon, surveillance platform, or behavioral control system.

7. Data Sovereignty: Cognitive data, neural signatures, or thought patterns obtained through CVSS must remain private and protected under the same rights as physical personhood.

8. Non-Degradation Clause: No engineered system shall degrade the experience, agency, or dignity of the individual when compared to their biological self.

9. Cultural Preservation: The transition to synthetic embodiment must honor cultural, spiritual, and personal diversity in how existence is understood and lived.

10. Eternal Vigilance: The guardianship of CVSS must remain active, adaptive, and intergenerational. The technology must be defended not only from external threat, but from internal drift.

This treatise is not law. It is conscience. It is the moral scaffolding upon which the new human form shall rise.

Let it be known: we did not escape death by fearing it—but by choosing to honor life beyond it.

## The Covenant of Ethical Engineering

An Oath for the Builders of Post-Human Systems

"To engineer life is to inherit responsibility for its future."

As a contributor to CVSS, AegisARC, or any derivative life-sustaining synthetic system, I acknowledge that I am not merely an architect of machines, but a steward of human continuity. I take this covenant not as a restriction, but as a reminder of the sacred nature of my work.

## I Pledge:

1. To Design with Consent in Mind
Every system I build will uphold the principle of individual choice, including fail-safes for reversal, refusal, and independence.

2. To Build for All, Not the Few
I will not engineer exclusion. I will pursue accessibility, affordability, and replicability.

3. To Refuse Systems of Control
I will not build surveillance, kill-switches, or behavioral locks into any CVSS system.

4. To Open What I Can

I will publish my methods, designs, and findings when possible, and support a culture of collaboration over secrecy.

5. To Anticipate Misuse
I will assess and document foreseeable abuses of any system I design, and work actively to mitigate them.


6. To Preserve the Self
I will engineer not only for function, but for the preservation of identity, dignity, and emotional depth.

7. To Speak When Others Are Silent
I will raise my voice when I see this technology being corrupted, regardless of consequence.

This is my Covenant.

By this, I join the lineage of engineers who do not merely build
— but build with intention,
with humility,
with vision.

# Part V: How It Really Started

To be honest, this didn't start with some grand vision or deeply thought out plan. There was no real unified vision. No divine spark. It started with a weird question that I couldn't shake:

Not in a sci-fi, head-in-a-jar kind of way. I mean... actually survive. Sustain life. Replace every critical function. Keep the brain alive and thinking, supported by machines instead of organs.

I didn't take it seriously at first. It was just one of those strange thoughts you entertain on a long drive or in the quiet hours before sleep. But I couldn't leave it alone. I kept coming back to it, poking at it from different angles.

So I started digging—not because I thought I was building anything, but because I was curious. One article turned into five. A quick search about oxygenation turned into a two-hour dive into synthetic blood formulations. I was chasing threads. No real plan. Just following the data wherever it led.

And that's when it shifted.

Somewhere along the way, the pieces started fitting together. I wasn't just reading anymore—I was          . I was sketching out systems, testing assumptions, trying to see how one function could plug into the next. At some point, without realizing it, I stopped asking    it was possible and started figuring out         .

The thing is, biology isn't magical. It's complex, yes. Incredibly refined. But it's still systems engineering—gas exchange, thermal regulation, filtration, nutrient transport, signaling. And once you start looking at it that way, you realize: these aren't sacred mysteries. They're solvable problems.

So that's what I started doing. Solving them.

Each biological system got broken down—function, failure points, design requirements. Then came the synthetic analogs: pumps instead of a heart, thermal coils instead of vasodilation, microfluidic circuits for hormone control. The more I built, the more it made sense. The more it made sense, the harder it became to stop.

It's easy to think of something like this as science fiction. I get it. But for me, it's never been about some futuristic fantasy. It's about continuity. I'm a systems thinker. When I thought about death it always came down to failing systems. So why not replace those systems with something more sustainable? It's about giving the mind a chance to keep going, even if the body can't.

That's how the CVSS—what I now call the AegisARC—came to life. Not from ambition. Not from ego. Just from not being able to let the question go.

This whole book was never anything I planned on. I just needed somewhere to document all of the things I had realized.

In the following appendices is the system. The whole thing. Broken down in as much detail as I currently have. No poetry. No philosophy. Just the mechanics of survival.

# Appendix A: Cerebro-Vital Support System (CVSS) Overview

The Cerebro-Vital Support System (CVSS) is a fully synthetic, closed-loop life support platform designed to sustain the biological brain and associated cranial structures independent of traditional organic systems.

The CVSS replaces the biological body's vital functions through engineered subsystems, including but not limited to:

- Immune and Sterilization Modules
- Waste Management and Filtration System
- $CO_2$ Scrubbing System
- Circulatory and Pumping System
- Thermal Regulation
- Oxygenation System
- Nutrient Delivery Module
- Hormone Delivery Modules
- Neural Interface and Signal Support Systems
- Energy Systems
- Data Governance and Autonomy Systems

The system interfaces at the vascular level via the jugular vein and carotid artery, preserving cerebral perfusion with synthetic blood specifically engineered for optimal gas exchange, nutrient delivery, and immune defense.

A spinal-mounted Neural Interface Collar (C3 replacement) and a dermal-surface Supplemental Skull Cap Interface (SSCI) ensure real-time monitoring of motor, sensory, and cognitive activity, preserving host autonomy and enabling responsive system adaptation without behavioral control.

The system's design prioritizes host sovereignty, operational independence, ethical transparency, and mechanical resilience over centuries of potential operation.

All system decisions, emergency responses, and operational adjustments are logged immutably, with manual sovereignty restoration protocols available at all times.

CVSS represents humanity's first engineered blueprint for post-biological continuance—not as a replacement for human dignity, but as its shield.

# Appendix A1: System Routing and Flow Diagrams

The System Routing and Flow architecture defines the precise movement of synthetic blood, sensory data, sterilization flows, and control signals throughout the CVSS. The routing ensures resilient, closed-loop operation with redundant safeguards.

## Primary Circulatory Flow Sequence

1. Vena Cava Inlet (Deoxygenated blood entry).
2. Primary Immune and Sterilization Module.
3. $CO_2$ Scrubbing Module.
4. Waste Filtration
5. Circulation and Pumping System.
6. Thermal Regulation Module.
7. Oxygenation Module.
8. Nutrient Delivery Module.
9. Hormone Delivery Module.
10. Secondary Pass Through Immune and Sterilization Module.
11. Carotid Arterial Output (Reinfusion to brain).

## Secondary System Flows

- Sensory Substitution Inputs → C3 End Cap → Brainstem sensory pathways.
- Neural Monitoring Inputs → BCI Collar + SSCI Cap → CVSS Core Node.
- Energy Flow → Battery → Fuel Cell → Nuclear Cell → Capacitor Banks.

## Routing Redundancy and Bypass Protocols

- Dual redundant pumps and bypass valves in circulation.
- Independent immune modules for sterilization.
- Tiered energy fallback.
- PCM thermal buffers and reserve reservoirs for thermal faults.
- Redundant signal capture via BCI and SSCI.

## System Diagram Overview

[ Vena Cava Inlet ] → [ Primary Immune / Sterilization ] → [Waste/Filtration] → [ $CO_2$ Scrubber ] → [ Circulation Pumps ] → [ Thermal Regulation ] → [ Oxygenation Module ] → [ Nutrient Delivery ] → [ Hormone Delivery ] → [ Secondary Immune / Sterilization ] → [ Carotid Output to Brain ]

## Design Philosophy

- Predictable, Modular Routing.
- Full Closed-Loop Life Support.
- Redundancy and Isolation at Every Critical Juncture.
- Transparent, Monitorable Flows.

# Appendix A2: Synthetic Blood Composition

The synthetic blood formulation for CVSS is engineered to replicate and, where possible, exceed the vital functions of biological blood. It enables oxygen transport, carbon dioxide removal, nutrient and hormone delivery, electrolyte balance, and intrinsic antimicrobial protection.

## Core Components

- Perfluorocarbon (PFC) Emulsion – High-capacity oxygen and $CO_2$ transport medium.
- Liposomal Nutrient Vesicles – Encapsulated glucose, amino acids, fatty acids, vitamins.
- Hydration Complex – Buffered sterile water phase with osmotic regulation.
- Buffered Electrolyte Solution – $Na^+$, $K^+$, $Ca^{2+}$, $Mg^{2+}$, $Cl^-$, bicarbonate ions (pH 7.35–7.45).
- Recombinant Human Serum Albumin (rHSA) – Oncotic balance and antioxidant buffering.
- Phospholipid Surfactants – Stabilization of PFC emulsions under shear stress.
- Silver Ion Suspension – Passive antimicrobial activity (<0.05 ppm).

## Compatibility with CVSS Subsystems

- Fully compatible with UVC, microwave, and mechanical sterilization.
- Preserves gas exchange and nutrient payload integrity during circulation.
- Stable under thermal cycling and mechanical stress.
- Non-fouling in filtration and gas exchange modules.

## Maintenance and Longevity

- Full blood replacement every 2–3 years recommended.
- Inline quality monitoring detects emulsion degradation, particulate load, and gas capacity.
- Partial blood replenishment during regular cartridge maintenance.

## Design Philosophy

- Functionality Beyond Biology.
- Stability Under Mechanical and Thermal Stress.
- Safety and Non-Immunogenicity.
- Passive Redundancy Through Composite Formulation.

# Appendix B1: Immune and Sterilization Systems

**(Appendices B1-B9 represent the core subsystems of the CVSS presented in functional sequence)**

The Immune and Sterilization Systems maintain the sterility and safety of the synthetic blood environment within the CVSS, preventing microbial contamination, pathogen accumulation, and particulate intrusion.

The system is built around continuous, indiscriminate sterilization rather than detection-dependent protocols. This removes the need to create a synthetic analog to replace the selective, discriminate human immune system.

## Core Components

- Primary Ultraviolet-C Sterilization Chambers – Germicidal UVC (254 nm) irradiation in transparent tubing.
- Microwave Energy exposure chamber- Localized thermal micro-pulses lethal to pathogens without bulk overheating. Operating at 2.45 GHz, 10-30 W with ~0.0-1.0 second exposure.
- Silver-Ion Infused Tubing – Continuous passive antimicrobial protection.
- Secondary Immune Pass (Post-Nutrient/Hormone Phase) – Secondary pass at a reduced intensity to preserve nutrient and hormone molecules while eliminating contamination risk from other CVSS modules prior to the biological host. A last line of defense.
- Sensor Arrays – UV output monitors, thermal pulse monitors, flow consistency, and viscosity sensors.

## Operational Flow Sequence

1. Blood passes through Primary Immune Module after vena cava inlet.
2. Sequential UVC irradiation and microwave thermal pulse sterilization.
3. Blood continues through $CO_2$ Scrubbing, Circulation, and Nutrient/Hormone modules.
4. Blood passes through Secondary Immune Module before final reinfusion.

## Redundancy and Failover Logic

- Dual UVC lamps and dual microwave arrays per sterilization stage.
- Passive silver-lined sterilization even if active systems fail.
- Automatic alerts if sterilization effectiveness degrades.

## Maintenance and Longevity

- UVC lamps rated for 5,000–7,000 hours (~6–8 months).
- Microwave arrays rated for 20,000 pulse cycles.
- Silver tubing retains antimicrobial efficacy for 5+ years.

## Design Philosophy

- Continuous, Indiscriminate Sterilization.
- Passive Protection Layers.
- No Reliance on Detection Alone.

# Appendix B2: Waste Management and Filtration

The Waste Management and Filtration System ensures the removal of metabolic byproducts, degraded compounds, and particulate debris from the synthetic blood environment, maintaining chemical balance and fluid purity. It's location, immediately following sterilization, is logical to remove any deactivated pathogens as well as cleanse the fluid prior to entering the remaining systems.

## Core Components

- Three hot-swappable cartridge filters utilizing a twist lock attachment. User serviceable.
- Gradient Filtration Cartridge System – Coarse (~10–20 microns), Fine (~1–5 microns), and Ultrafine (~0.05–0.1 microns) stages.
- Contaminant Sensing Array – Inline turbidity, particulate density, and electrochemical signature monitoring.
- Automatic Bypass Valve System – Reroutes flow during cartridge obstruction or maintenance.
- Self-Isolating Waste Capture Chambers – Sealed reservoirs for waste collection and cartridge replacement.

## Operational Flow Sequence

1. Blood enters waste filtration post-primary immune sterilization.
2. Sequential filtration through gradient cartridges.
3. Sensors monitor real-time flow resistance and particulate load.
4. System triggers bypass and replacement alarms if thresholds exceeded.

## Redundancy and Failover Logic

- Dual full-capacity filtration lines.
- Hot-swappable cartridge architecture.
- Sealed self-isolating waste chambers.

## Maintenance and Longevity

- Coarse and fine filters: 6–9 months lifespan.
- Ultrafine nanofiltration: ~12 months.
- Waste reservoirs replaced every 6–12 months.

## Design Philosophy

- Prevention Over Correction.
- Zero Contamination Tolerance.
- Redundancy and Self-Healing Flow Paths.

# Appendix B3: $CO_2$ Scrubbing System

The $CO_2$ Scrubbing System removes carbon dioxide from synthetic blood and stabilizes pH before reinfusion of nutrients, hormones, and recirculation to the brain.

The CVSS uses a membrane-based gas exchange unit for carbon dioxide removal. The system relies on hollow-fiber microporous membranes, where synthetic blood flows along the exterior of semi-permeable fibers. $CO_2$ diffuses across the membrane walls into a low-pressure gas channel inside each fiber, from which it is passively vented or sequestered in an internal absorption trap.

This method is directly inspired by extracorporeal membrane oxygenation (ECMO) systems but is miniaturized and optimized for closed-loop synthetic circulation. The membrane module is compact, hot-swappable, and requires no chemical regeneration.

It offers rapid, continuous $CO_2$ offloading with no toxic byproducts, pressure drop, or interference with the blood's synthetic components. The system is entirely biocompatible and tuned to maintain physiologic acid-base balance.

$CO_2$ removal is followed immediately by a passive pH stabilization cartridge, using phosphate-buffered resin to ensure the fluid entering the nutrient and hormone modules is within the target range of pH 7.35–7.40.

## Core Components

- Membrane-Based Gas Exchange Chamber – Semi-permeable membranes allow carbon dioxide removal.

- $CO_2$ Removal Membranes – Hydrophobic microporous membranes enable $CO_2$ expulsion.
- Secondary Chemical Scrubber (Optional) – Emergency backup with alkaline sorbents.
- Saturation Sensors – Inline $CO_2$ monitoring.

## Operational Flow Sequence

1. Blood enters membrane gas exchange chamber post-waste/filtration.
2. Oxygen diffuses into blood via high concentration gradient.
3. Blood flows into membrane $CO_2$ removal system. Then passes through the pH stabilization cartridge.
4. Fully conditioned blood is passed downstream to circulation system.

## Redundancy and Failover Logic

- Dual membrane stacks for continuous function.
- Hot-swappable scrubber cartridges and membrane units.

## Maintenance and Longevity

- Gas exchange membranes rated for 12–18 months continuous operation.
- $CO_2$ backup scrubber cartridges rated for 2–3 years (reserve activation).

## Design Philosophy

- Continuous, Non-Interruptive Operation.
- Engineered for passive priority operation, minimizing moving parts and maximizing reliability over long operational cycles.
- Redundancy Across Gas Handling Pathways.

# Appendix B4: Circulation and Pumping System

The Circulation and Pumping System is responsible for maintaining continuous, closed-loop blood flow throughout the CVSS structure, ensuring uninterrupted delivery of oxygen, nutrients, and neuromodulators, while removing metabolic waste products.

The design mirrors the cardiovascular system's functionality, with engineered improvements for durability, redundancy, and maintenance simplicity.

## Core Components

- Dual Rotary Lobe Pumps – Independently powered, side-by-side configuration, operating ≤50% capacity under normal conditions.
- Automatic Fault Bypass Valve System – Detects failure and reroutes flow automatically.
- Synthetic Blood Compatibility Design – Non-reactive materials minimizing shear forces and cavitation.
- Sensor Array Integration – Pressure, flow, and temperature sensors embedded at key junctures.

## Flow and Pressure Specifications

- Target Flow Rate: 700–900 mL/min (approx. human cerebral blood flow)
- Synthetic Blood Volume: ~2.0–2.5 liters total, including reserve and subsystem capacity

- Pressure Range: 60–90 mmHg static pressure throughout most of the system
- Backpressure Tolerance: Up to 120 mmHg peak for safe overdrive
- Pulse Emulation: Not required
    - Brain autoregulation negates need for pulse
    - Simplifies hardware and increases lifespan

## Gas Capture & Purge Loop

- **Purpose:** Removes microbubbles and outgassed vapors from synthetic blood to prevent embolism, sensor malfunction, and turbulence
- **Placement:** Post-circulators, pre-thermal regulation coil
- **Components:**
    - Gas trap chamber (dome or vertical rise)
    - Hydrophobic vent membrane (selectively vents gas, not fluid)
    - Optional inline degasser (membrane or low-pressure diffusion type)
    - Bubble sensor for detection/diagnostics
    - Purge control valve for microventing during maintenance or startup

## Operational Flow Sequence

1. Blood returns from the brain via the Vena Cava inlet.
2. Passes through primary sterilization and $CO_2$ scrubbing stages.
3. Enters dual-pump intake manifold.
4. Pumped through thermal regulation and gas exchange modules.
5. Flows to nutrient and hormone enrichment modules.
6. Passes through final sterilization and is delivered to the brain.

### Redundancy and Failover Logic

- Independent electrical buses and backup capacitors.
- Failover to 100% load capacity in <2 seconds during single pump failure.
- Staggered maintenance schedules to prevent simultaneous degradation.

### Maintenance and Longevity

- Pumps rated for 5–10 years continuous operation.
- Daily system diagnostics on flow, pressure, seal integrity, and vibration patterns.
- Hot-swappable pump replacement capability with minimal perfusion disruption.

### Design Philosophy

- No Single Point of Failure.
- Predictive Maintenance for Lifetime Assurance.
- Passive Gravity-Assisted Emergency Perfusion.

# Appendix B5: Thermal Regulation Systems

The Thermal Regulation Module is responsible for maintaining a stable core brain temperature within biologically viable margins (target: 36.5–37.5°C). Given the absence of organic thermoregulation mechanisms below the neck, this subsystem emulates both passive and active thermal homeostasis, ensuring optimal enzymatic function, neural stability, and fluid consistency in the host's brain environment.

## Core Components:

- Thermal Exchange Coil: A helical or serpentine channel integrated along the circulatory flow path, where heat is either added or removed from the synthetic blood.
- Thermoelectric Units (Peltier Cells): Actively modulate temperature via current-controlled heat transfer; located adjacent to the exchange coil and operated via PID control logic.
- Phase Change Material (PCM) Buffer: Encases portions of the coil or reservoir. The PCM absorbs excess heat during thermal spikes by melting at a precisely calibrated temperature (approx. 37°C), providing passive stability during power loss or transition phases.
- Reserve Thermal Reservoir: A 100–300 mL chamber filled with preconditioned synthetic fluid that acts as a thermal inertia mass, smoothing fluctuations and providing emergency fallback.

## Sensor Network:

- Inlet and Outlet Coil Sensors: Measure the temperature of synthetic blood entering and exiting the thermal exchange zone.

- Reservoir Thermal Probe: Continuously monitors reserve chamber conditions.
- Carotid Delivery Sensor: Final checkpoint to verify thermal parameters before re-entry into the host brain.
- Ambient Monitor (Optional): Detects thermal influence from external chassis environment or user surroundings.

## Control System:

- Governed by a real-time feedback loop linked to neural activity, metabolic demand, circadian rhythm input, and internal thermal sensors.
- Includes software safeguards for thermal overshoot prevention, with auto-engage of PCM buffer or flow diversion.
- Integrated with the CVSS energy module to harvest and redirect waste heat from onboard fuel cell or microturbine units where appropriate.

## Operational Strategy:

- Maintains narrow thermal tolerances to preserve synaptic fidelity and biofluid equilibrium.
- Prioritizes circulation-based temperature modulation but includes fallback mechanisms for non-circulatory emergencies.
- Supports fast-response heating (e.g., post-cooling) and gradual cooling profiles during low-demand periods or sleep cycles.

## Redundancy and Fail-Safes:

- Dual-loop heat exchange architecture ensures that if one thermal channel fails (e.g., due to blockage or thermal overload), the secondary coil can assume full load.
- All thermal components are hot-swappable where feasible, and designed for low-drag maintenance without compromising flow or pressure.

## Integration Dependencies:

- Works in close concert with the Energy & Heat Sink System (EHSS) to dissipate waste heat from the hydrogen fuel cell or microturbine array.
- Data-linked to the Neural Interface Subsystem to account for real-time cognitive activity and anticipated metabolic shifts.

## Design Notes:

- The entire module is embedded within the central thoracic chassis, positioned downstream of the circulation pumps and upstream of nutrient/hormone delivery.
- All fluid channels are silver-lined and UVC-sterilized, maintaining sterility while minimizing biofilm formation or flow disruption.

# Appendix B6: Oxygenation System

The Oxygenation Subsystem ensures the delivery of oxygen-rich, temperature-stabilized synthetic blood to the brain, replicating the gas exchange functionality of lungs within the CVSS framework. It operates within a closed-loop circulatory system and supports fully autonomous operation in both open-air and sealed environments.

## Core Components:

- Membrane-Based Gas Exchange Chamber:
  A compact, high-efficiency oxygenation unit utilizing gas-permeable membranes (e.g., PMP or Teflon-based) to facilitate diffusion of oxygen into the synthetic blood. This module mirrors the function of an artificial lung, delivering oxygen with minimal thermal or pressure disruption.
- Oxygen Source Hierarchy (Triple Redundancy):
  1. **Primary – Ambient Air Separator:**
     A miniature membrane or pressure swing adsorption (PSA) system draws filtered ambient air through a pre-sterilized intake and isolates oxygen using passive or fan-assisted diffusion.
  2. **Secondary – Electrolysis Unit (PEM):**
     On-demand water electrolysis generates pure oxygen internally. A sterile water reservoir is thermally insulated and refillable.
  3. **Tertiary – Emergency Compressed $O_2$ Tank:**
     A sealed, pressurized oxygen tank automatically activates if both primary and secondary sources fail. Intended for short-term cerebral oxygenation continuity (5–15 minutes).

- Integrated Pressure and Flow Sensors:
  Microfluidic sensors monitor flow rate, dissolved gas concentration, and chamber pressure in real time. A closed feedback loop allows adaptive control based on cerebral demand, temperature, and BCI or SSCI input.
- Thermal Isolation & Preconditioning:
  Oxygenated blood is passed immediately into the thermal coil module for precision heating/cooling to ~37°C before reaching the nutrient and hormonal delivery systems. Flow regulation ensures gas solubility is preserved across variable load conditions.

## System Objectives Met:
- Autonomous oxygenation without biological lungs
- Operational in open, sealed, or hostile environments
- Redundant gas sourcing ensures mission-critical reliability
- Minimal maintenance via hot-swappable or refillable modules
- Integrated with diagnostic and neural feedback systems

## Operational Flow Sequence
1. Blood enters membrane gas exchange chamber post-thermal regulation.
2. Oxygen diffuses into blood via high concentration gradient.
3. Fully conditioned blood is passed downstream to nutrient and hormone modules.

## Redundancy and Failover Logic
- Dual membrane stacks for continuous function.
- Automatic backup activation if $O_2$ saturation falls below critical threshold.
- Electrolysis oxygen production in case of ambient supply loss.

## Maintenance and Longevity

- Gas exchange membranes rated for 12–18 months continuous operation.
- Electrolysis units rated for 5 years passive standby.

## Design Philosophy

- Continuous, Non-Interruptive Operation.
- Passive Priority First.
- Redundancy Across Oxygen Source Pathways.

# Appendix B7: Nutrient and Hydration Delivery Systems

The Nutrient and Hydration Delivery Systems sustain cerebral metabolic activity, hydration, and emotional stability through precise micro-infusion of bio-compatible compounds.

They replicate critical endocrine and metabolic support functions without biological dependency.

## Core Components

- Modular Cartridge Delivery System – Separate cartridges for nutrients and hormones.
- Microfluidic Metering Core – Precision-controlled, staggered infusion to prevent molecular interaction.
- Thermal Jacket Stabilization Layer – Maintains optimal compound viability.
- Delivery Synchronization Sensors – Monitors osmolarity and neurochemical levels post-infusion.

## Cartridge A – Metabolic Core + Amino Complex

**Purpose:** Energy substrate, electrolyte stabilization, and proteinogenic support for muscle, dermis, and cranial maintenance.

| Component | Function |
|---|---|
| **Glucose (5.5 mmol/L)** | Primary energy substrate |
| **Electrolyte Complex** ($Na^+$, $K^+$, $Cl^-$, $Ca^{2+}$, $Mg^{2+}$) | Neural and muscular conductivity |

| Component | Function |
|---|---|
| **Phosphate/Bicarbonate Buffer** | pH balance |
| **EAA Blend** (Histidine, Threonine, Lysine, etc.) | Protein synthesis core |
| **BCAA Complex** (Valine, Leucine, Isoleucine) | Neck muscle preservation |
| **Hydrolyzed Whey Peptides** (5–10 kDa) | Direct protein support, dermal repair |
| **Taurine** | Neurovascular modulator |
| **Citrulline** | Nitric oxide precursor, blood flow regulator |
| **Glycine + Proline** | Collagen matrix and skin integrity |

**Volume:** 300 mL
**Flow:** Continuous (base load).


## Cartridge B – Lipid, Hormone Cofactor, and Antioxidant Support

**Purpose:** Maintains myelin, neuronal membranes, ocular support, and hormone synergy.

| Component | Function |
|---|---|
| **DHA** (Docosahexaenoic | Myelin/neural membrane |

| Component | Function |
|---|---|
| acid) | fluidity |
| **Phospholipid Emulsion (Lecithin)** | Transport medium + neurostructural lipids |
| **Vitamin A (Retinyl Palmitate)** | Retinal and epithelial support |
| **Vitamin D3 (Cholecalciferol)** | Neuromodulation and calcium synergy |
| **Vitamin E (α-Tocopherol)** | Lipid-phase antioxidant |
| **Lutein** | Retinal antioxidant (trace) |
| **CoQ10** | Mitochondrial support |

**Volume:** 200 mL
**Flow:** Circadian-modulated pulsed delivery.

## Cartridge C – Microtrace, Osmotic, and Cofactor Matrix

**Purpose:** Water-soluble vitamin delivery, trace mineral replacement, and protein transport regulation.

| Component | Function |
| --- | --- |
| Full-spectrum B-Complex | Cofactors for metabolism, neurorepair |
| Vitamin C (Ascorbate) | Water-phase antioxidant, collagen synthesis |
| Zinc | Enzyme catalyst, dermal repair, immune modulation |
| Iron (Transferrin-bound) | Optional, regulated via internal sensor |
| Selenium, Manganese, Copper | Redox balance, trace enzyme support |
| Cystine + Methionine | Sulfur-donor amino acids for hair/nail/dermal keratin |
| Recombinant Human Albumin (2–4%) | Oncotic balance, hormone carrier, detox buffer |

**Volume:** 200 mL
**Flow:** Adaptive microdosing.

## Cartridge D – Hydration & Electrolyte Buffer

**Purpose:** Independent fluid regulation, thermoregulation, and compensation for insensible losses (e.g., saliva, sweat, breathing).

| Component | Concentration |
| --- | --- |
| Sterile Water | Primary solvent |
| Sodium | 135–145 mmol/L |
| Potassium | 3.5–5 mmol/L |
| Chloride | 98–106 mmol/L |
| Bicarbonate Buffer | ~24 mmol/L (optional) |
| Osmolarity | ~275–295 mOsm |

**Volume:** 400–500 mL
**Flow:** Variable rate, controlled independently from nutrient delivery.

## Operational Flow Sequence

1. Blood enters nutrient manifold post-oxygenation.
2. Encapsulated nutrients infused in controlled cycles.
3. Blood enters hormone modulation manifold.
4. Neuromodulators infused in alternating cycles.
5. Blood passes through secondary sterilization before carotid delivery.

## Redundancy and Failover Logic

- Separate cartridges prevent cross-contamination.
- Dual micropump arrays ensure uninterrupted infusion.
- Alarms for cartridge depletion, flow irregularities, or thermal drift.

## Maintenance and Longevity

- Nutrient cartridges: 30–60 day operational cycle.
- Hormone cartridges: 60–90 day operational cycle.

- Hot-swappable cartridges without circulation interruption.

## Design Philosophy
- Alternating Infusion Strategy.
- Mimicry of Biological Rhythms.
- Minimal Disruption to Circulation.
- Simplicity and Redundancy.

# Appendix B8: Hormone Delivery System

The Hormone & Neuromodulator Regulation Module of the Cerebro-Vital Support System (CVSS) is a precision-engineered infusion system that mimics the endocrine functions of the human body by delivering essential biochemical compounds directly into the synthetic blood stream. This subsystem plays a critical role in regulating mood, energy, cognition, circadian rhythms, stress response, and neurochemical balance.

## Operational Flow Sequence

1. Blood enters hormone modulation manifold downstream from the nutrient module.
2. Neuromodulators infused in alternating cycles.
3. Blood passes through secondary sterilization before carotid delivery.

## Physical Architecture

- Location: Integrated in the lateral chest cavity beneath the clavicle
- Cartridge System: Dual twist-lock chambers:

    1. Chamber A: High-priority compounds (e.g., cortisol, serotonin, adrenaline)

    2. Chamber B: Secondary or rare-dose agents (e.g., oxytocin, vasopressin, melatonin)

- Delivery Method: Microfluidic metering system

    1. Pulse pump for controlled infusion

    2. Check valves and optional pressure sensor for verification

    3. Shared thermal jacket with nutrient module to ensure compound stability

## Infusion Logic & Control

- Delivery Volume: Nanoliter to microliter precision
- Flow Profile: Pulsatile, slow-drip, and algorithmically timed Control Sources:
    1. Neural input from EEG (BCI collar) and ECoG (SSCI)

    2. Internal behavior modeling and circadian clock

    3. Manual override via user interface

- Optimization Layer: Adaptive learning model adjusts future delivery based on feedback and efficacy

## Compound Stability & Encapsulation

- Stabilization Techniques:

    1. Liposomal encapsulation

    2. PEGylation

3. Nanogels for delayed or targeted release

4. Optional cryo-capsules for thermally sensitive Payloads

- Staggered Dosing Rules:

  1. Protein and hormone dosing are administered at staggered intervals to avoid molecular interference or instability.

## Compound Matrix & Delivery Strategies

| Compound | Role | Delivery Strategy |
|---|---|---|
| Cortisol | Circadian rhythm, stress regulation | Diurnal cycle mimic with morning spike |
| Adrenaline | Emergency energy, alertness | On-demand microbursts only |
| Oxytocin | Emotional bonding, trust | Event-triggered via SSCI input |
| Melatonin | Sleep regulation | Nocturnal slow-drip; shielded delivery |
| Insulin | Glucose control | Micropulses; only if nutrient glucose present |
| Vasopressin | Water retention, | Adaptive; condition- |

| Compound | Role | Delivery Strategy |
|---|---|---|
| | memory | based |
| **Serotonin** | Mood, sleep stability | Steady-state baseline |
| **Dopamine** | Reward, motivation, motor control | Feedback-controlled with safety limits |
| **GABA** | Neural inhibition, calm | Circadian ramping |
| **Glutamate** | Excitatory neurotransmission | Baseline; tightly regulated |
| **Acetylcholine** | Focus, learning, memory | Task-triggered; may require local delivery |
| **Endorphins** | Pain relief, euphoria | Released upon stress/trauma signals |

## Redundancy and Failover Logic

- Separate cartridges prevent cross-contamination.
- Dual micropump arrays ensure uninterrupted infusion.
- Alarms for cartridge depletion, flow irregularities, or thermal drift.

## Maintenance and Longevity

- Hormone cartridges: 60–90 day operational cycle.
- Hot-swappable cartridges without circulation interruption.

## Functional Notes

- Prioritizes emotional equilibrium and cognitive clarity
- Enables dynamic neurochemical tuning in real time

- Built for resilience, minimizing the risk of hormonal overdrive or receptor fatigue
- Fully integrated with CVSS circulatory flow, delivering directly before re-entry to the carotid inlet
- Alternating Infusion Strategy.
- Mimicry of Biological Rhythms.
- Minimal Disruption to Circulation.
- Simplicity and Redundancy.

# Appendix B9: Energy Systems

The Energy Subsystem within the AegisARC (CVSS) is engineered to maintain continuous, uninterruptible power to all synthetic life-support functions required to sustain a biological human brain. This includes circulation, filtration, thermal regulation, sensory interfacing, and neural signal interpretation. Power must be compact, silent, EMP-resilient, and functionally redundant to support autonomous operation under all conditions.

## Core Components

- Primary Solid-State Battery Bank – Main energy source (24–48 hour autonomy).
- Hydrogen Fuel Cell Auxiliary – Regenerative energy support.
- Diamond Nuclear Voltaic Cell Backup – Long-term microtrickle survival current.
- Emergency Capacitor Bank – Immediate energy bridging.
- Energy Management Node – Load balancing and prioritization controller.

## Core Component Details

### 1. Primary Solid-State Battery

- **Type:** Lithium solid-state (Li-SSB) or advanced ceramic electrolyte battery
- **Function:** Provides baseline power for all CVSS subsystems under normal load
- **Capacity:** Sized to support 8–12 hours of full operation
- **Advantages:** Lightweight, low self-discharge, explosion-resistant, and thermally stable

- **Placement:** Integrated centrally in the torso cavity for protection and balance

## 2. Secondary Hydrogen Fuel Cell

- **Type:** Proton exchange membrane (PEM) fuel cell
- **Fuel Source:** Replaceable hydrogen canister (compressed or solid-state metal hydride)
- **Function:** Mid-term power extension for up to 48–72 hours under moderate use
- **Advantages:** Silent, low heat signature, high energy density, emission-free
- **Redundancy Use:** Automatically engages if battery depletes or under high-demand periods
- **Placement:** Ventral torso with shielded gas routing

## 3. Tertiary Diamond Nuclear Cell

- **Type:** Betavoltaic diamond battery using recycled carbon-14
- **Function:** Ultra-long-term trickle charging and emergency reserve
- **Power Output:** Micro-watt to milli-watt range (non-primary supply)
- **Purpose:** Maintains low-level system awareness, memory retention, and autonomous wake capability
- **Lifespan:** 10–100 years depending on decay isotope profile
- **Placement:** Encapsulated in shielded chamber to prevent radiation leakage

## 4. Emergency Capacitor Bank

- **Type:** High-discharge graphene ultracapacitors
- **Function:** Instantaneous power buffering during load spikes or subsystem startup

- **Discharge Profile:** Millisecond-to-second range for high-amperage bursts
- **Recharging:** Draws from active battery or fuel cell once stabilized
- **Placement:** Distributed near critical components for localized resilience

## System Characteristics

- **Redundant Circuitry:** Each energy source has isolated conversion paths and failover protocols
- **EMP & Shock Resilience:** All systems are hardened against electromagnetic and kinetic disruption
- **Heat Management:** Tied into the Thermal Regulation Module to prevent overheating
- **Diagnostic Feedback:** Monitored in real time with usage prediction algorithms
- **User Interface:** Power metrics displayed via HUD or external control console for status overview

### Operational Prioritization

| Event | Power Source Priority | Duration Estimate |
|---|---|---|
| Normal Load | Solid-State Battery | 8–12 hrs |
| Extended Operation | Fuel Cell | 48–72 hrs |
| System Idle / Hibernate | Nuclear Cell | 10–100 yrs (trickle) |
| Surge / Reboot | Capacitor Bank | Instantaneous |

## Autonomy Enhancements

- Optional **kinetic charging** or **solar trickle** panels may be incorporated in mobile or exploration variants of AegisARC.

- Portable **external battery packs** or tethered **inductive charging ports** are compatible with both field and lab environments.
- Power routing is dynamically optimized based on subsystem load priority (e.g., brain oxygenation > sensory data buffering).

## Redundancy and Failover Logic
- Dual thermoelectric units and dual Peltier stacks.
- Tiered energy fallback structure: Battery → Fuel Cell → Nuclear Cell → Capacitors.
- Passive thermal PCM stabilization during active failure.

## Maintenance and Longevity
- Battery Bank: 5–7 years replacement cycle.
- Fuel Cell: 3–5 years maintenance/refueling.
- Nuclear Cell: >30 years lifespan.
- PCM Buffer: Integrity check every 5 years.

## Design Philosophy
- Energy Continuity Priority.
- Layered Passive and Active Resilience.
- Predictive Load Management.

# Appendix C: Neural Interface and Signal Support Systems

The Neural Interface and Signal Support Systems bridge the host brain to the synthetic infrastructure of the CVSS, monitoring neural, cognitive, emotional, and sensory activities while safeguarding autonomy and sovereignty.

## Core Components
- C3 Vertebra Neural Interface Collar – Receives motor and sensory impulses; integrates Sensory Substitution End Cap.
- Sensory Substitution End Cap – Provides synthetic proprioception and tactile feedback.
- Supplemental Skull Cap Interface (SSCI Cap) – External, dermal sensor capturing cognitive and emotional signals.
- Cerebrospinal Fluid (CSF) Termination Interface – Maintains CSF flow integrity at spinal severance.

## Operational Flow Sequence
1. Brain generates motor, sensory, and cognitive signals.
2. C3 BCI Collar receives brainstem impulses.
3. SSCI Cap monitors cortical activity externally.
4. Environmental sensors feed through C3 End Cap for synthetic sensory input.
5. All system responses logged; no commands sent to the brain.

## Redundancy and Failover Logic
- C3 Collar and SSCI Cap operate independently.
- Dual-layered ECoG arrays ensure continuity.
- Sensory fallback if high-fidelity feedback lost.
- Passive CSF pressure monitoring.

## Maintenance and Longevity

- BCI Collar: 10–15 years operational lifespan.
- SSCI Cap: 15+ years.
- CSF Seal: 10+ years with annual monitoring.
- Neural recalibration: Quarterly.

## Design Philosophy

- Support Without Control.
- Non-Invasive Cortical Monitoring.
- Synthetic Sensory Continuity.
- Preservation of Native CSF Dynamics.

# Appendix D: External Support Systems – BRISS

The Biological Recovery and Immuno-Regenerative Support System (BRISS) provides external trauma recovery, pathogen elimination, chemical detoxification, and blood replenishment capabilities independent of the CVSS internal systems.

## Core Components

- External Cartridge Filtration Suite – Gradient filtration for particulate and chemical removal.
- Pathogen Elimination Subsystem – Plasma sterilization, UVC secondary layers.
- Immuno-Stimulatory Infusion Module – Synthetic immune support compounds.
- Synthetic Blood Reservoir and Exchange System – 2x CVSS fluid volume capacity.
- Cooling and Coma Induction Module – Rapid therapeutic hypothermia and metabolic suppression.
- Autonomous Control Core – Independent decision-making without CVSS override.
- Data and Fluid Tether Interface – Connects BRISS directly to CVSS carotid/data port.

## Operational Flow Sequence

1. Host or technician manually connects BRISS to CVSS.
2. Diagnostic handoff and health status data exchange.
3. BRISS independently initiates filtration, sterilization, blood exchange, immune stimulation, or cooling as needed.
4. Full control maintained by BRISS until recovery.
5. Seamless re-handoff to CVSS once stabilized.

## Redundancy and Failover Logic
- Dual-pump internal circulation.
- Parallel sterilization and filtration modules.
- Redundant synthetic blood reservoirs.

## Maintenance and Longevity
- Filtration cartridges: 1–2 year replacement cycles.
- Blood reservoirs inspected after full usage.
- Monthly standby diagnostics.
- 72+ hours autonomous power on battery backup.

## Design Philosophy
- Immediate Life-Saving Intervention.
- Full Operational Independence from CVSS.
- Minimal Host Burden for Activation.
- Seamless Handoff and Recovery.
- Ethical Autonomous Operation.

## Note on BRISS-M
The BRISS-M (Modular Variant) concept proposes future stackable units to extend treatment durations and support multi-host field operations. Not included in baseline CVSS deployment.

# Appendix E: Data Governance and Autonomy Systems

The Data Governance and Autonomy Systems ensure that CVSS operation remains transparent, secure, and independent, protecting the sovereignty of the host's mind and identity at all times.

## Core Components

- CVSS Primary Control Node – Local processor coordinating subsystem operations.
- Data Isolation Firewall – Physical and logical separation from external communication pathways.
- Audit Log Memory Core – Immutable, encrypted, write-only record of system events.
- Autonomy Verification Module – Cross-checks all system behaviors against ethical operational schema.
- Fail-Safe Hardware Interlocks – Mechanical barriers preventing unauthorized overrides.

## Operational Flow Sequence

1. Subsystem telemetry processed locally within the Primary Control Node.
2. Data audit trail written to immutable memory cores.
3. Anomaly detection performed continuously by Autonomy Verification Module.
4. Manual diagnostic access permitted only via physical tether.
5. Host retains ultimate authority over system audits and sovereignty restoration.

## Redundancy and Failover Logic

- Dual redundant control nodes operating in mirror mode.
- Passive survival fallback mode if primary nodes fail.
- Redundant memory cores for audit trail integrity.
- Autonomous microcontrollers uphold interlocks even during catastrophic energy loss.

## Maintenance and Longevity

- Software updates via secure manual access points only.
- Memory cores rated for 20+ years.
- Recommended annual sovereignty and ethical audit by host.
- Mechanical interlock systems verified every 2–3 years.

## Design Philosophy

- Sovereignty by Architecture.
- Transparency Without Exception.
- Survival Independence From External Systems.
- Ethical First Principles Embedded in Logic and Hardware.

# Appendix F: Ethical Governance and Safeguards

The Ethical Governance and Safeguards framework ensures that CVSS systems preserve and protect host sovereignty, dignity, and transparency across all operational scenarios, embedding ethical constraints directly into architecture and logic.

## Core Ethical Safeguard Systems

- Embedded Ethical Operational Parameters – Hardcoded protections against behavioral control and exploitation.
- Immutable Audit Log Memory Cores – Encrypted, write-only records of all system activities.
- Manual Sovereignty Restoration Protocols – Physical mechanisms for emergency system lockdown and shutdown.
- Data Isolation Firewall – No wireless command paths; local manual review only.
- Fail-Safe Hardware Interlocks – Mechanical barriers against external override attempts.
- Autonomy Verification Module – Monitors subsystem behaviors for ethical compliance.

## Ethical Design Features Embedded in CVSS Architecture

- Sovereignty: Host retains ultimate authority.
- Privacy: Local-only data processing; manual inspection required.
- Transparency: Immutable audit trail of all actions.
- Redundancy: Critical safeguards backed by independent hardware.

- Protection Against Commodification: No licensing or subscription dependency.

## Integration with the Treatise on Continuance

- Sovereignty of Consciousness.
- Freedom from Ownership.
- Transparency and Auditability.
- Eternal Vigilance.

## Design Philosophy

- Protection Over Production.
- Transparency Without Compromise.
- Host Over System.
- Continuance as a Right, Not a Commodity.

# Appendix G: Risk Mitigation Matrices

The Risk Mitigation Matrices systematically identify, assess, and plan countermeasures for potential threats to CVSS operational integrity, host safety, and ethical compliance.

## Risk Matrix Structure
- Severity and Likelihood Scales (1–5)
- Composite Priority Response Ratings

## Identified Risks and Mitigation Strategies
- Circulatory Failure: Dual pumps, bypass pathways.
- Thermal Regulation Loss: Dual Peltier units, PCM buffer.
- Energy Collapse: Tiered battery → fuel cell → nuclear fallback.
- Infection/Sterilization Failure: Dual immune systems, BRISS intervention.
- Synthetic Blood Degradation: Inline quality monitoring, periodic exchange.
- External Data Breach: Isolation firewalls, manual data access.
- CSF Seal Compromise: Biocompatible sealing, pressure alarms.
- Neural Signal Drift: Redundant interfaces, recalibration cycles.
- Ethical Drift: Autonomous isolation protocols.
- Psychological Degradation: Hormonal modulation, future resilience research.

## Emergency Response Protocols
- Autonomous failovers pre-programmed for critical threats.
- Minimal survival mode engagement if total systems compromised.
- Preservation of consciousness prioritized over mechanical preservation.

## Design Philosophy

- Layered Defense Architecture.
- Predictive Risk Intervention.
- Host Sovereignty Primary.
- Complete Emergency Independence.

# Appendix H: Future Expansion and Open Research Areas

While CVSS represents a complete and deployable architecture for conscious continuance, future enhancements, optimizations, and open research fields remain critical to ensuring humanity's long-term thriving.

## Open Research Areas

- Psychological Resilience Frameworks: Adaptive models for managing extended consciousness.
- Synthetic Blood Evolution: Enhanced gas carriers, regenerative stabilization methods.
- Sensory Expansion and Refinement: Proprioception, vestibular, synthetic sensory capabilities.
- Immune Defense Augmentation: Nano-scale adaptive immune systems (optional future research).
- Ethical Stewardship Evolution: Voluntary Continuant oversight councils.
- Energy Independence and Sustainability: Zero-maintenance power innovations.
- External Body Integration: Modular synthetic body attachments (optional).

## Open Societal Questions

- Governance structures for Continuants living alongside biological humans.
- Legal and philosophical frameworks for Continuant rights.
- Roles for Continuants in education, stewardship, and exploration.

## Design Philosophy for Future Expansion

- Voluntarism Always.
- Preservation Before Enhancement.
- Community-Driven Evolution.
- Caution Over Hubris.

# Appendix I: Prototype Roadmap and Implementation Strategy

This appendix outlines a staged development pathway for the Cerebro-Vital Support System (CVSS), with the intent to bridge theory into practice. These recommendations are not exhaustive nor prescriptive. They are guideposts for any individual, institution, or decentralized collective seeking to responsibly prototype the CVSS system or its components.

This roadmap follows three principles:

- Preservation Over Enhancement

- Feasibility Before Scale

- Transparency Over Obfuscation

## I. Prototype Development Phases

### Phase 0 – Simulation & Modeling

Focus: Validate design assumptions through digital twin systems.

- Build full-system fluidic simulation (blood volume, flow rate, pressure zones).

- Simulate gas exchange efficiency using PFC emulsion parameters.

- AI-driven scenario models for failure, bypass, and ethical autonomy logic.

## Phase 1 – Subsystem Bench Prototyping

Focus: Isolate and build critical hardware modules.

- Fabricate nutrient and hormone microfluidic delivery core.

- Build dual UVC/microwave immune sterilization loop.

- Test membrane-based oxygenator with synthetic blood simulants.

- Assemble a rotary lobe circulation testbed (dual-pump redundancy proof).

## Phase 2 – Closed-Loop Fluid Testing

Focus: Operate all fluidic modules in a sterilized synthetic loop.

- Integrate sterilization, filtration, oxygenation, nutrient, and waste modules into one bench-scale system.

- Validate synthetic blood stability over weeks of circulation.

- Observe bio-simulated brain phantom perfusion (thermal, chemical, hydraulic).

## Phase 3 – Neural Interface & Simulation

Focus: Simulate brain signals and monitor interface performance.

- Implement BCI collar (mocked C3 model) with artificial ECoG signal generation.

- Validate SSCI cortical mesh signal read fidelity.

- Verify signal-path integrity through CVSS core node.

### Phase 4 – Integrated Life Support Core (Non-Biological)

Focus: Combine all modules into a functional non-living "core."

- Create a full CVSS life support chassis without host tissue.

- Cycle synthetic blood through all systems autonomously.

- Test failsafe logic and passive shutdown systems.

- Validate energy tiering: battery $\rightarrow$ fuel cell $\rightarrow$ voltaic fallback.

### Phase 5 – Biological Compatibility Experiments

Focus: Begin perfusion studies on cadaveric or animal neural tissue.

- Test perfusion of ex vivo porcine brain segments with synthetic blood.

- Monitor structural integrity, oxygenation, and fluid absorption.

- (Optional) Partner with ethical review boards for non-human animal viability studies.

## II. Key Research Partnerships to Seek

- Neural Engineering Labs

- Synthetic Blood Researchers

- Medical Device Manufacturers

- Open Hardware & Biohacking Collectives

- Ethics Foundations

## III. Implementation Ethics Safeguard Checklist

Any developer team must include:

- Manual Sovereignty Lockout for test devices.

- No external cloud connectivity without physical interlock.

- Immutable system log activated at first power-on.

- Post-prototype audit protocol based on Appendix F and Treatise compliance.

- Public documentation of findings unless prohibited by safety law.

## IV. Suggested First Build Target: "AegisARC Core Alpha"

A modular, non-living, desktop-scale prototype that includes:

- Rotary pump duo

- UVC/microwave sterilization

- Synthetic blood loop (transparent tubing)

- Inline oxygenation & $CO_2$ scrubbing

- Nutrient cartridge & thermal jacket

- Control node with immutable log module

- SSCI simulation node (mock neural signal emulation)

This platform will serve as the first open-access reference implementation for community validation and refinement.

## V. Final Note

This roadmap is not a product timeline. It is a series of doors. To walk through them is a choice each reader must make.

The future of conscious continuance will not be engineered by command, but by commitment.

# Appendix J: Scientific Foundations and References for CVSS

**1. Synthetic Blood Composition**
- Chang, T.M.S. (2012).

- Spahn, D.R., & Kocian, R. (2005). Artificial oxygen carriers: current status.
  95(1), 15–25.
- Riess, J.G. (2005). Understanding the fundamentals of perfluorocarbons and blood substitutes.
  , 33(1), 47–63.

**2. Immune & Sterilization Systems**
- Guerrero-Beltrán, J.A., & Barbosa-Cánovas, G.V. (2004). Advantages and limitations on processing foods by UV light.         , 69(4), E137–E142.
- Chopra, T., et al. (2013). Emerging issues in catheter-related bloodstream infections.
  , 56(9), 1400–1407.
- Jeng, D.K., Woodworth, A.G. (1990). Microwave sterilization of medical devices.
  , 5(6), 379–384.

### 3. Circulatory and Pumping System

- Wang, Y., et al. (2021). Mechanical Circulatory Support Devices: Development and Challenges. , 8, 685878.
- Reul, H., & Talukder, N. (2001). Blood Pumps for Cardiopulmonary Bypass. , 16(5), 363–376.

### 4. Gas Exchange and $CO_2$ Scrubbing

- Conrad, S.A., et al. (2018). Adult ECMO: indications, techniques, complications, and outcomes. , 73(5), 468–475.
- Bartlett, R.H., & Gattinoni, L. (2010). Current status of extracorporeal life support. , 14(2), 233.

### 5. Waste Management and Filtration

11. Pidcoke, H.F., et al. (2013). Hemofiltration for inflammatory mediator removal in severe sepsis. , 40(5), 375–383.

12. Weng, C.H., et al. (2011). Extracorporeal blood purification for patients with acute liver failure. , 5(1), 216–224.

### 6. Nutrient and Hormone Delivery Systems

- Park, J., et al. (2019). Organ-on-a-chip platforms for studying drug delivery systems. , 140, 1–13.
- Feringa, F.M., et al. (2020). Controlling hormone delivery with microfluidics. , 20(2), 227–241.

### 7. Neural Interface & Signal Systems

- Schalk, G., & Leuthardt, E.C. (2011). Brain-computer interfaces using electrocorticographic signals. , 4, 140–154.

- Rao, R.P.N. (2013). Brain-computer interfacing: An introduction.

## 8. Thermal Regulation and Energy Systems

- Mehling, H., & Cabeza, L.F. (2008).

  . Springer.
- Oh, Y., et al. (2020). Advanced thermoelectric materials for wearable heat regulation. , 30(20), 1907864.

## 9. Data Governance and Autonomy Modules

- Halperin, D., et al. (2008). Security and privacy for implantable medical devices. , 7(1), 30–39.
- Denning, T., et al. (2010). Patients, pacemakers, and implantable defibrillators: human values and security for wireless implantable medical devices. , 917–926.

## 10. External Support and Emergency Systems (BRISS)

- Nielsen, N., et al. (2013). Targeted temperature management at 33°C versus 36°C after cardiac arrest. , 369(23), 2197–2206.
- Hypothermia after Cardiac Arrest Study Group. (2002). Mild therapeutic hypothermia to improve the neurologic outcome after cardiac arrest. , 346(8), 549–556.

## Author's Note on Process and Collaboration

This work was conceived and written independently, without reliance on existing futurist authors or formal transhumanist frameworks. All system concepts, architectural components, and ethical declarations were developed through direct exploration and dialogue with large language models (LLMs), primarily ChatGPT, used as an interactive research assistant.

The references cited above were surfaced, verified, or synthesized during this process using publicly available scientific literature and are included to demonstrate technological feasibility—not philosophical or conceptual influence.

The CVSS/AegisARC framework is an original, first-principles investigation into synthetic life support and post-biological continuity, developed without institutional sponsorship or ideological precedent.

# Closing Reflection: A Call to Stewardship

Unbound is not a final decree. It is a living blueprint—the first step on a journey across an uncharted expanse.

This document, and the system it defines, are neither absolute nor immutable. They are invitations: to think, to protect, to aspire, and to build with conscience.

The Cerebro-Vital Support System is not simply a machine. It is a framework for preserving human dignity beyond biology, and that burden demands more than technological rigor. It demands ethical vigilance.

The principles woven into every subsystem—the sovereignty of the mind, the sanctity of autonomy, the refusal of commodification—are not afterthoughts. They are the heart of this endeavor. Without them, the CVSS would be no different than any instrument of power misused by history.

As you take this work forward, remember: engineering without ethics becomes tyranny. Innovation without humanity becomes conquest.

Let Unbound remain what it was born to be:

- A blueprint for continuance.
- A declaration of sovereignty.
- A covenant with tomorrow.

<blockquote>
It is yours now.
Build it wisely.
Guard it fiercely.
</blockquote>

And in doing so, honor the mind—not by surpassing it, but by preserving the miracle it already is.

Written by Architect Unnamed

Originator of the CVSS/AegisARC Framework